Dash Diet Super Guide for Weight Loss

How to GUARANTEE Weight Loss with the Dash Diet

By: Amy Weis

I0435222

PUBLISHERS NOTES

Trade Paperback Edition

Manufactured in the United States of America

WHAT YOU WILL LEARN IN THIS BOOK
How This Book Will Help You and Why

The Dash Diet is one of the many diets that you hear and read about daily. The truth is that there is merit in most of these diet programs but they are only a part of the solution to the problem of weight gain and obesity. It is only by going on a real diet that addresses all of the problems that lead to diseases such as diabetes, binge eating and bulimia.

This book will guide you through the process of how to get the most out of the Dash Diet and almost guarantee success!

ABOUT THE AUTHOR

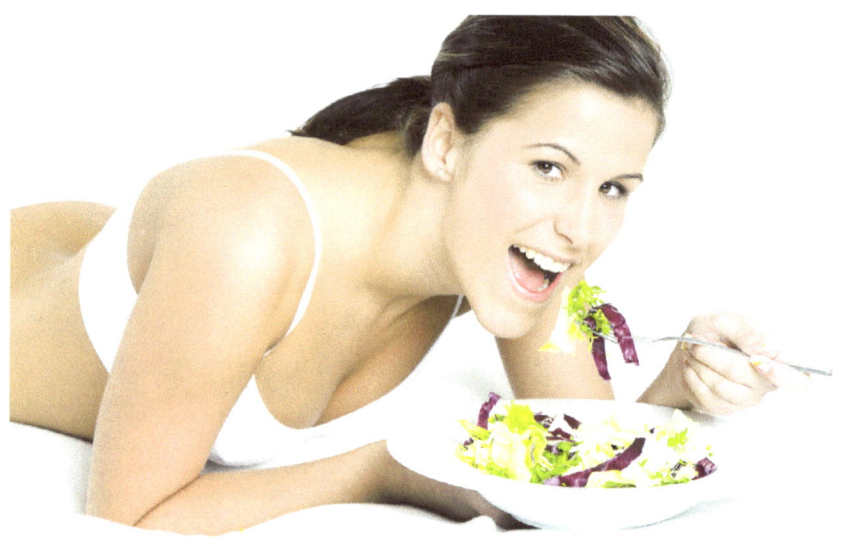

Amy struggled for months with her weight problem after the birth of her first child. She tried every diet you can think of and none seemed to deliver one that would allow her to eat healthy for her new born and more importantly helped to keep the weight off.

She eventually found the Dash Diet which was never meant for Mums trying to lose the baby fat but was really for hypertensive adults. She took the Dash Diet and made it her own. Everyone she has helped so far has been successful using her strategies and pointers.

Now you too can use Amy's tips in this guide to blow it out of the water with this diet!

TABLE OF CONTENTS

DEDICATION

"Your diet is a bank account. Good food choices are good investments."

- Bethenny Frankel

INTRODUCTION - WHY WE ENDORSE THE DASH DIET

The DASH diet – which stands for Dietary Approaches to Stop Hypertension – is aimed squarely at the epidemic of high blood pressure and heart disease in the United States. It's not a weight-loss diet; instead, it's an approach to lifelong eating that may cut your risks of osteoporosis and cancer along with cardiovascular problems.

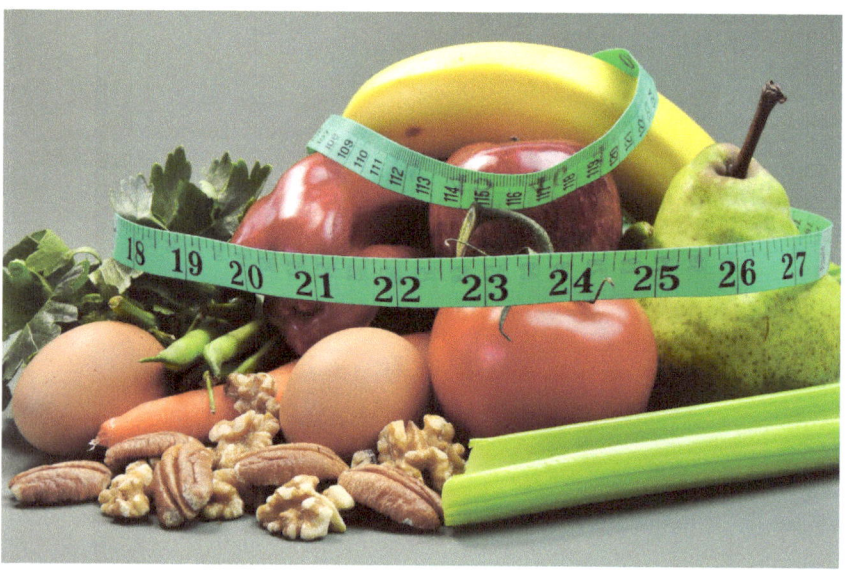

By following the DASH diet for two weeks, you potentially can shave a few points off your blood pressure and start to lower your risks of complications from hypertension. If you follow the program for months, you may be able to bring your blood pressure down to normal levels, especially if it's not extremely high to start.

Salt in Diets Contributes to Hypertension

Approximately one-third of all adult Americans suffer from high blood pressure, defined as a pressure above 120 systolic and 80 diastolic and usually written as 120 over 80, or 120/80. Prehypertension is defined as a blood pressure between 120/80 and 139/89. Any pressure above that is defined as hypertension, which may require drug treatments as well as dietary interventions.

Doctors consider sodium to be a major cause of hypertension, and the DASH diet was developed primarily to restrict salt content in a daily diet. Most Americans eat far too much sodium every day – nearly twice the daily recommendation of 2,300 milligrams per day.

DASH Cuts Daily Sodium Intake

When following the DASH diet, you need to keep your sodium intake below 2,300 milligrams. If your doctor recommends following the modified lower sodium DASH diet, you'll be consuming no more than 1,500 milligrams of sodium per day. This may seem like a drastic cut in sodium from what you normally eat, but believe it or not, you can accomplish it mainly by cutting out high-sodium processed foods.

Which foods have too much sodium? Processed meats, canned soups and vegetables – unless they're marked "low sodium" – contain too much for the DASH diet. You also should steer clear of salted crackers and chips. It's possible to find low-salt versions of most of these foods.

Diet Guidelines for DASH Program

In addition to cutting salt, the DASH program calls for you to eat specific amounts from various food groups.

For example, you should get six to eight daily servings of grain products – preferably from whole grain sources, such as whole wheat or brown rice. The diet also calls for four to five servings of vegetables, including healthy choices such as carrots, sweet potatoes and greens. Fruits – fresh, frozen or canned – should make up another four to five servings.

Look for two to three servings daily of low-fat or fat-free dairy products, including milk and yogurt. And try to get six or fewer servings of meat – only lean meat, including skinless chicken and fish and occasional lean beef – per day to meet your protein requirements. When consuming oil, keep it to a minimum, and choose only heart-healthy oils such as olive oil.

When following the DASH diet, its okay to slip up occasionally; as long as you follow the diet fairly faithfully long-term, you should begin to see results in the form of lower blood pressure.

Would you prefer not to have to count calories when you diet? What about high-protein, high-fat and low-carbohydrates as a diet? Do you know the difference between low-fat and low-carbohydrate foods? And why is some fat in your food good for you?

And why does sugar appear in so many foods nowadays? Not just in soda but also peanut butter! In fact, are low-fat processed meals good for you at all? And what about "cheat days" and "binge eating" - why are they harmful to your diet? Can you drink wine or beer when you diet? Can you lose weight if you always eat out? You will be surprised at what we suggest.

And how many calories do you need to eat a day in order to lose weight? What is your Body Mass Index (BMI) and what should you do about it? How often should you weigh yourself? The answers to these questions may surprise you.

All of these questions, and more, are answered in this book. You will find helpful advice in the answers to assist you in going in the real DASH DIET.

Before you begin the DASH Diet you need to follow these guidelines and follow our suggestion to really make the program work wonders in your life and make you ten times healthier that you were before.

We have spent a LONG time researching answers to your most burning dieting questions.

The information supplied is based on the latest current medical understanding of how our bodies absorb the foods we eat and what strategies we should follow if we want to shed unwanted weight.

The most important thing is that you need to be happy about what you are eating, and you need to learn about portion-size control for yourself.

And exercise is strongly recommended – not just because turning fat into muscle makes you look thinner, although that is a good thing (muscle has greater density than fat, so 1 kilo of muscle is smaller than 1 kilo of fat). We cannot recommend an exercise plan for you as it depends upon what you want to do. You do not need to go to a gym or get a personal trainer, though. You can jog around your local park, take up cycling, and go swimming regularly. Just be active.

It is easy to measure weight, just jump on the bathroom scales, but what about fat? Fat around the thighs or buttocks seems to be less of a health risk to that on the waist.

The recommendation is to have a waist-size (measured at the tummy button) equivalent to less than half you height. Whilst losing weight, you want to retain as much muscle as you can. One of the questions describes metabolism and the importance of keeping your muscle bulk as you age. It is a real aid to weight loss.

So stop reading this section and get straight on to the questions and their answers. You will not be disappointed.

DASH DIET SUPER GUIDELINES

DO I HAVE TO EXERCISE OR JUST STICK TO THE DASH DIET ALONE?

We often hear that a little exercise is a key to weight loss. For example, use the stairs instead of taking an elevator. But research shows that it is better to cut down our calorie intake.

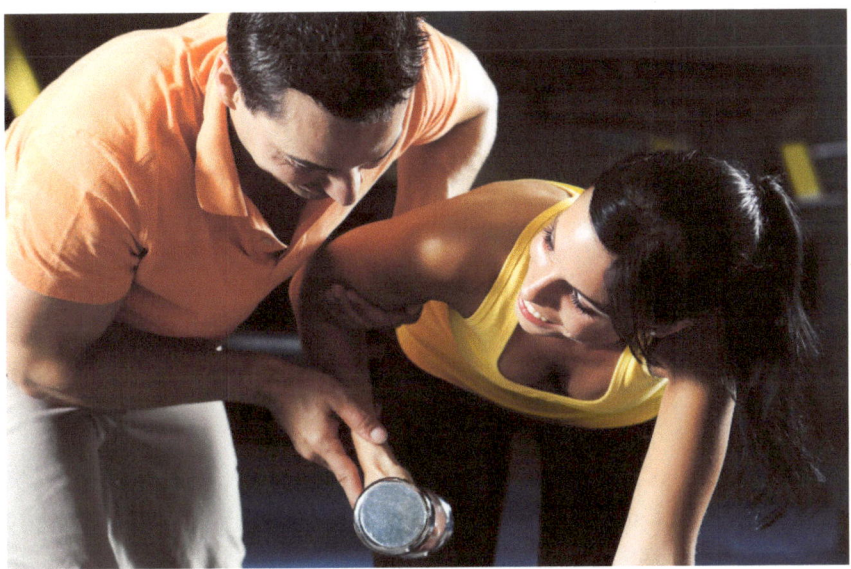

To achieve a 300 calories energy deficit, you can run in the park for 3 miles, or not eat 2 ounces of potato crisps (or chips). Studies that compare exercise with dieting show that participants tend to lose weight by dieting alone than by exercise alone. Both together are even better as they work in harmony.

Exercise has effects on hunger and appetite hormones. These make you feel noticeably hungrier after exercise. If you walk briskly for an hour and burn 400 calories, and then have a slice of pizza with some beer as the exercise made you hungry, you will eat more calories than you burned off. It may not be pizza with beer, but people do often naturally compensate for calories burned.

For every action there is a reaction, we learn in physics, but this law seems to work in biology too. Our body has compensatory mechanisms to counteract the effect of exercise. When we exercise a lot and get tired, we may well rest for the remainder of the day. Some of the calories we burn come from our normal movements during the day.

So if you become tired after exercise and then sit on the couch for the rest of the day, you may well lose the energy deficit gained from the exercise.

TO LOSE WEIGHT, HOW MANY CALORIES DO I HAVE TO BURN?

While the Dash Diet does not focus on calorie counting you need to expend more calories per day than you eat, for your body to lose weight.

Your body has a base metabolic rate (BMR), which equates to a set number of calories a day. If you eat more calories than your body needs, you will gain weight. Many studies have found that in general women need 1,500-2,000 kcal to maintain their current weight and for men the range goes to 2,000-2,500 Kcal.

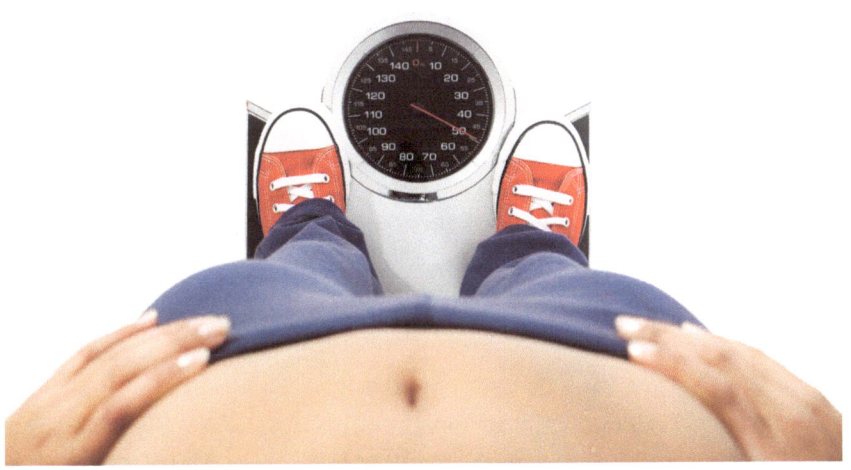

If you consistently eat fewer calories than your body needs in a day, it will start to convert body fat into energy to keep going. If you starve yourself long enough, your body will start using its own muscle fibre as an energy source. Remember that you use energy to digest food. So you have to be balanced about thinking of calories alone.

Remember that 1 pound of fat = 3,500 calories approximately. This means that if you consume 3,500 more calories than what you burn in a period of time you will gain one pound in weight. But if you manage to burn 3,500 more calories than you consume you will lose 1 pound in weight.

So to lose weight, you need to eat fewer calories than your body needs to run itself, OR increase your BMR by exercising more. But be careful... Not eating enough during the day slows down your metabolism two ways.

First, your body thinks it's starving, so it will slow down your calorie-burning capacity in order to "survive." Second, you are likely to make up for low-caloric intake in the last few hours of the day, causing your body to hang on to the food through the night in preparation for another day of "starving."

DO I NEED TO USE A BMI CALCULATOR WHEN ON THE DASH DIET?

While this is not really spoken about on the Dash Diet using the BMI calculator can definitely help during the weight loss process.

The Body Mass Index (or BMI) is a way of seeing if your weight is appropriate for your height. The actual calculation is your weight (in pounds) divided by your height (in inches). BMI is divided into several categories, and generally the higher you're BMI, the greater your risk of a large range of medical problems.

The chart below indicates the weight in pounds and height in feet and inches. For example if an individual is 180 cm in height **(Approximately 5 feet & 9 inches)** and weighs 63 Kilograms (**About 140 pounds)**; the BMI is 20.1 which is considered normal.

On the other hand, if the same individual weighs 86 Kilograms (**just about 190 pounds**), the BMI is 27.1 and the person is referred to as being overweight while a BMI of 34.4 for the same individual (with a weight of 240 pounds) is considered obese.

Body Mass Index

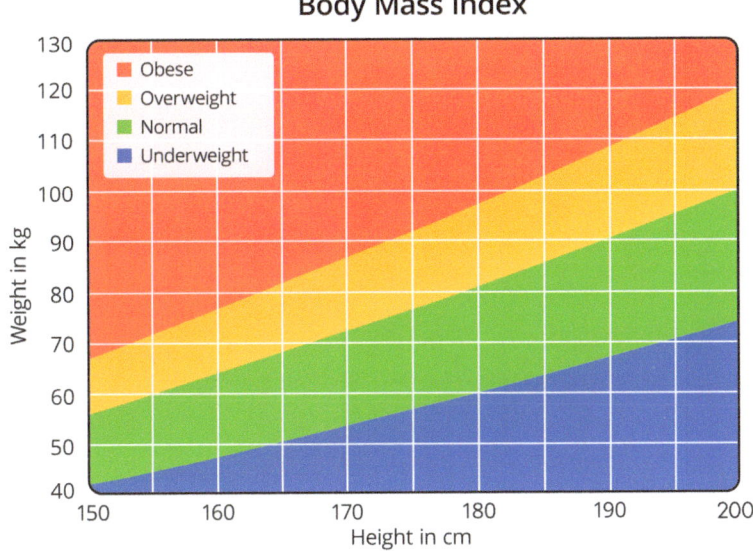

If the same individual has a weight of 120 pounds, the BMI is 17.2 and the person is said to be underweight. You can easily determine your BMI if you know your weight and height.

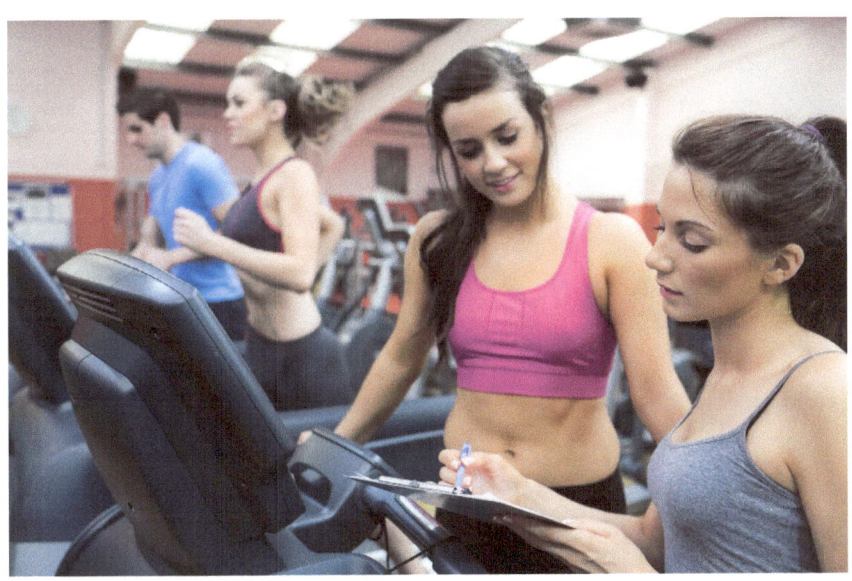

BMI charts are calculated for adults only. There are separate charts available for children's weight and heights. Inaccuracies can occur if you are an athlete or very muscular as this can give you a higher BMI even if you have a healthy level of body fat and the adult BMI chart is not appropriate for women who are pregnant or breastfeeding, or people who are very frail.

As BMI is based on weight and height, by losing weight you will reduce your BMI and put yourself into a lower risk group. A healthy diet, including a balance of food groups, vitamins and minerals, is essential for a long and active life. Keeping it simple, body weight and shape are a balance of energy intake (dietary calorific content) against output (calorific burn from activity & exercise).

IS IT HARDER TO LOSE WEIGHT WITH THE DASH DIET AS YOU GET OLDER?

As a general rule as someone gets older, the body loses some lean muscle mass every year. The rate is about 2-3% per decade. With the loss of muscle, it becomes harder to lose weight, as your metabolism slows down. "Metabolism" is a word for the chemical reactions that occur in your body to keep it alive, conversion of food into energy and building materials.

WHAT DOES METABOLISM SLOWING DOWN HAVE TO DO WITH DIETING?

Metabolism is a word for the chemical reactions that your body undergoes to keep it alive. The process of metabolism is what allows you to grow and eventually have children. Your body has a basal metabolic rate (BMR) - the rate at which these processes occur. You might have a high BMR (which allows you to lose weight easily) or a low BMR (which makes you gain weight). The BMR is determined by many factors, and the most important ones are your age, your sex, your height, your body weight, and your activity level.

Metabolism is like all chemical processes and slows down as you age. Your BMR slows down due to the loss of lean muscle mass, which makes it difficult for you to lose weight. The decrease may be 2-3% with each decade. In women, oestrogen levels drop after menopause. This drop causes thyroid hormones that regulate metabolism to drop too.

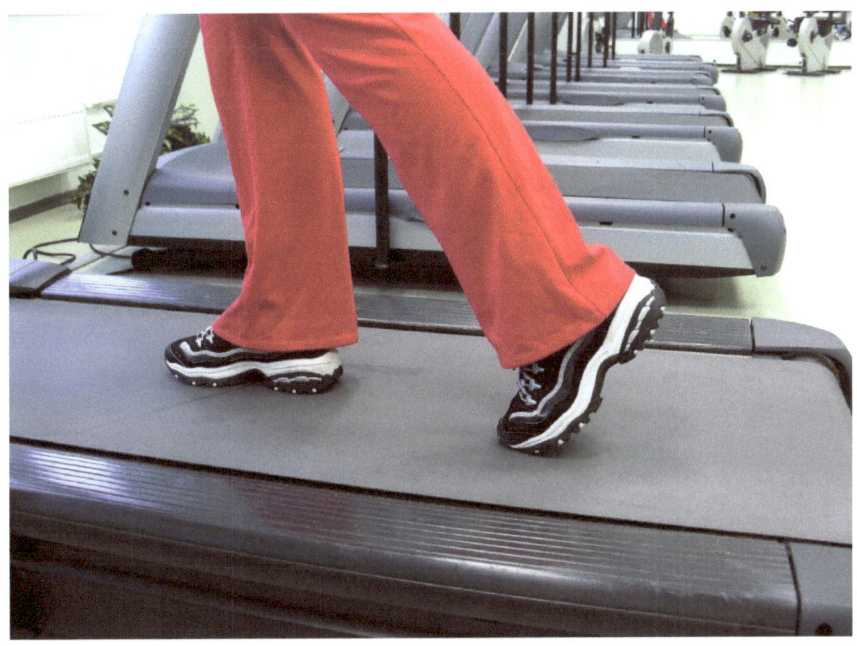

As your BMR slows down, your body burns fewer calories than before, and this can lead to weight gain if you do not cut down your calorie intake as well.

DOES THE DASH DIET WORK FOR MEN MORE THAN WOMEN?

Men and women have many different physical characteristics. Men are usually more muscular than women. Muscles burn more energy than body fat.

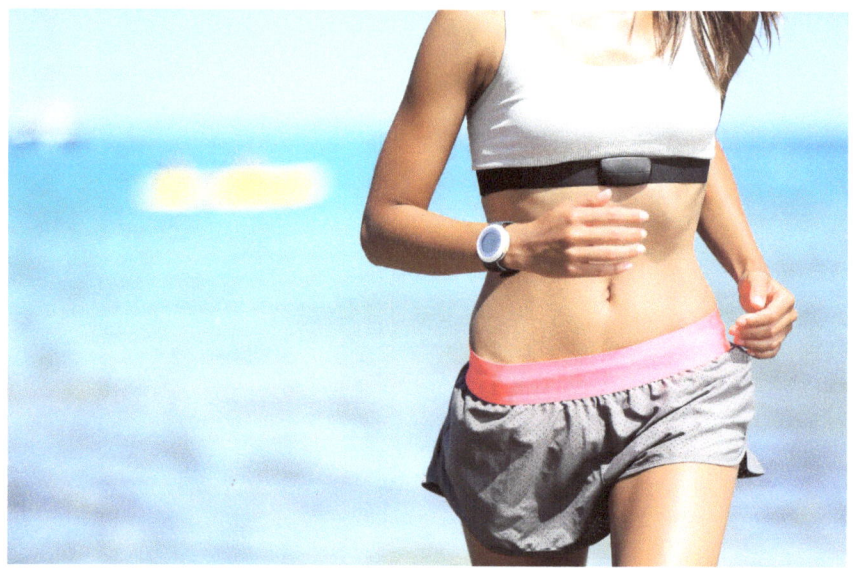

Women are predisposed to store and retain fat. Women have higher levels of oestrogen, a hormone that works to keep the fat on a woman's body so it's easier for her to get pregnant. That means women have to work harder to lose weight at the same rate as men.

Men's bodies respond more quickly to exercise. Women's bodies, meanwhile, actually go into a sort of starvation mode, slowing the metabolism to hang onto more fat.

Women may have a lower tolerance for exercise. Women have smaller lung capacity than men, which can make women feel as though they are working harder than men even if the women are working at the same level. This can also make exercise feel harder in high heat or humidity conditions.

What can I do about food craving when I am on the Dash Diet and how can I stop it?

Distractions – "If only chocolate will do", is a craving, not hunger. Cravings usually last about ten minutes. Recognize that and distract yourself: phone someone, make some tea, listen to music, sing, run an errand, or simply exercise.

Destroy the temptation – If you have given in and bought a box of chocolates or biscuits, and feel guilty when eating them, destroy them. Pour water or something else over them to make them uneatable. Do not think about the money you are wasting. If the chocolates or biscuits do not go into the rubbish bin, they are going onto your hips or tummy.

Be nutty - Drink two glasses of water and eat an ounce of nuts (for example 20 peanuts). Within 20 minutes, this will extinguish your craving and dampen your appetite.

Avoid triggers – Change what you eat. The longer you avoid your trigger foods, the less likely you may be, to want them. In fact, you may begin to crave the foods you DO eat on your diet.

Reduce your stress levels - Since cravings can be brought about by stress, learning to deal with stress could potentially save you hundreds of calories a day. This takes some effort and may require you to learn some techniques to manage your stress.

Avoid or Plan - Vary your usual routine so you don't normally walk past the bakery, or pizza restaurant. If you know you will be face-to-face with some cake at work, build a portion into the day's calories for your diet.

IF I CUT CARBOHYDRATES COMPLETELY FROM MY MEAL PLANS, CAN IT HARM ME, IS IT UNHEALTHY?

The Dash Diet does not say that you should remove all carbs from your diet but if you cut carbohydrates out of your diet for a couple of weeks, you will lose weight. It is one of the best ways to lose weight. Without insulin, your body will lose weight very easily. The only foods that make your body produce insulin are carbohydrates – this is why cutting out carbohydrates can have such an amazing effect.

To have maximum impact you probably want to do the first stage of the Atkins diet (remember we said a combination of all diet types is always best). This allows for no more than about 20 grams of carbohydrates each day - so this would allow you a small portion of green vegetables or salad with each of your main daily meals and NO other carbohydrates. No pasta, bread, potatoes, coloured vegetables, fruit, rice, etc.

Your body burns carbohydrates for energy. Depriving it of carbohydrates forces it to turn to fat for fuel – which is a state called "ketosis". If you follow a very low- or no-carbohydrate diet you might lose more weight than on a low-fat diet since you are eating less overall. Researchers have not yet determined the long-term effects of ketosis on human health. It is possible that this IS a very healthy way of eating, as opposed to cutting, say, all fat from your diet.

If I eat at night; can it hurt my Dash Diet Plan?

When you eat a meal late at night, it does not permit the body to be active enough to burn off the calories you have eaten within a few hours of finishing the meal. Health experts suggest that going to bed soon after eating means that more calories are converted to fat. They suggest you stay up for at least two or three hours after a meal, and one hour after a snack.

Additionally, staying up should mean maintaining some level of activity, not slouching in front of the TV. Sitting in a recliner chair is the same as going into the bed. The recliner is where a lot of people tend to get into trouble, as there is a tendency to relax at the end of the day, and to indulge in snack foods. If you stay up very late, a snack at midnight is fine, as long as you plan it into the overall daily calorie schedule, and that you stay up for long enough to digest it. The best thing is to eat healthy snack, a carrot or a cucumber will do just well.

I am on diet, how often should I weigh myself?

It is generally recognised that a weekly weighing is best. Doing it daily can cause "scale obsession" whereby you become obsessed with how much you weigh.

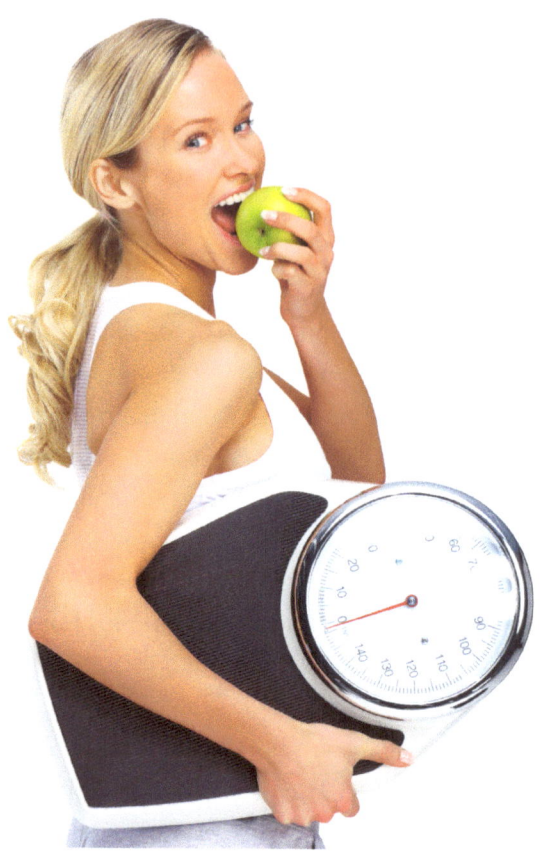

With things like water retention, weight can vary by as much as five pounds throughout the day, so it is vital that you weigh yourself at the same time each time you get on the scales to get a meaningful figure. Weighing yourself weekly does not give the same gratification as weighing yourself each day but it does mean you actual progress downwards to your goal weight can be very pleasing.

If you start to see that your dieting effort is paying off, it can be very motivating. Without the constant daily nag of the scales, you can have more of a worry-free diet and feel less pressured. You can concentrate on the diet, and be more at ease when you eat. If you have a slip up one day, there is still time to recover before the scales hand down their next judgement.

So weigh yourself at the same time each week, for example, on a Saturday morning, before you eat anything.

CAN I TAKE SUPPLEMENTS WHEN ON THE DASH DIET TRYING TO WEIGHT LOSS?

Are there weight loss supplements that are safe and helpful during the Dash diet? The following is a list of products you can get from some health food or pharmacies that have some weight-loss evidence behind them:

Green tea extract

Meal replacements

Calcium

Fibre

Conjugated linoleic acid (CLA)

Please remember to check with your doctor before taking any type of supplement. Supplements can have side effects and may interfere with any medications you take. And, when it comes to weight loss, there are no quick fixes. Only healthy eating and exercise have been proven to result in weight loss.

That is why dieters are recommended to focus on eating low-calorie foods that have bulk like whole fruits and vegetables, in addition to grains and low-fat dairy and meat. Also, start a fitness program and start to move about more - standing more, taking the stairs, or walking. Change your environment, too, so that it is supportive of a healthy lifestyle - keep fresh fruit in your office, plan meals, and take your lunch to work with you.

CAN I DRINK ALCOHOL WHEN ON THE DASH DIET?

Alcohol contains what are known as "empty calories". They do not contribute anything worthwhile to your body's need for nutrients. So it is best to cut down or eliminate all alcohol from your diet when trying to lose weight. Use those calories for foods your body REALLY needs.

Drink alone does not cause a "beer belly", but there are links between alcohol and fat metabolism.

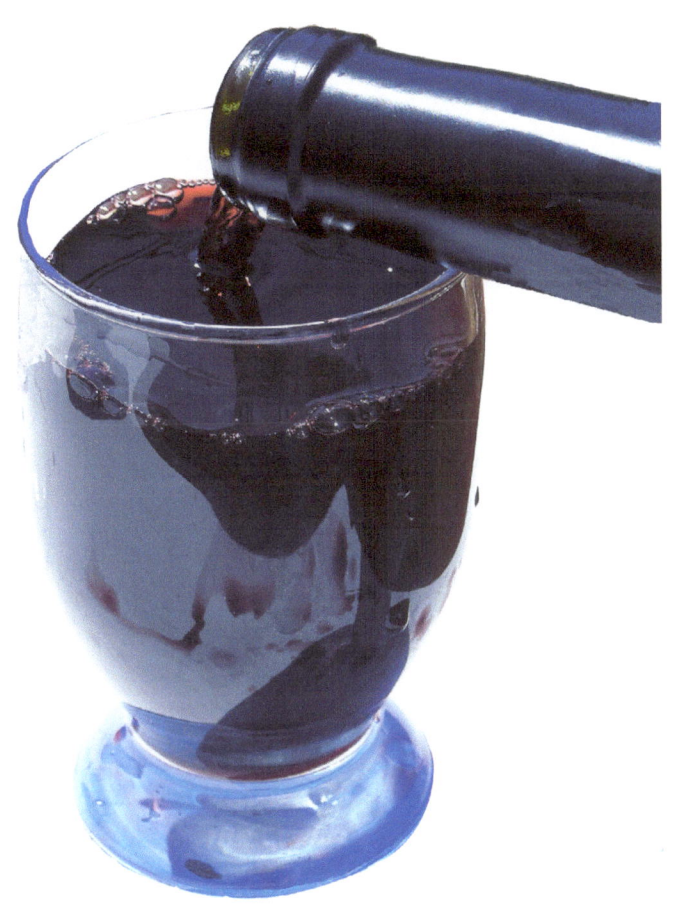

When you drink alcohol, your liver slows down its conversion of fat and carbohydrates into energy to eliminate the "dangerous" alcohol in your bloodstream first of all.

If you burn more calories than you eat or drink, you will lose weight. And while alcohol on its own will not inhibit weight loss unless you drink too much too often, drinking alcohol can have a negative result on your chances of eating properly, sleeping well and leading a healthy life style.

WHAT CAN I EAT WHEN I'M OUT ON THE DASH DIET?

Yes, you can if you follow these suggestions.

Beware of "light" dishes. More and more restaurants are promoting low-calorie, healthy choices, but, unfortunately, the claims are not always true. Read the menu carefully. Look for a mix of lean protein (fish, chicken breast, pork tenderloin, strips of steak), complex carbohydrates (brown rice, whole wheat pasta) and mono-unsaturated fats (canola or olive oil). If you need more information to help you choose the healthiest meals, go to the restaurant's website ahead of time to check if they list nutritional information for each dish they serve.

Don't be afraid to ask. Restaurants will try and meet all kinds of special requests - all you have to do is ask. Ask for your food to be grilled (or baked, broiled, poached, or steamed) instead of fried. Ask for dishes to be cooked with some olive oil instead of butter.

Practice portion control. Eat three-quarters of what is on your plate and then stop. This simple step can easily shave up to 300 calories off your meal. What is more, you will be satisfied from eating 75 percent of your dinner, and you will barely miss those extra few bites.

Be smart about salad. At the salad bar, fill your plate with vegetables, greens, chickpeas, and Japanese edamame, and top it with one or two tablespoons of low-fat dressing. Skip the bacon lardons, cheese, bread croutons, and creamy dressings, and the pasta, tuna, or chicken salads swimming in mayonnaise. If you can't resist, restrict yourself to JUST a quarter-cup serving.

Pick the right protein. So you must have steak? A 10-ounce rib-eye can be 700 calories or more. Instead, order a leaner cut of beef, such as tender-loin, flank steak, or strip. The recommended serving size is approximately 5 ounces (you can measure this as being approximately the size of the palm of your hand). If the restaurant does not offer one that small, cut your portion in half and take the uneaten part home (in a doggy bag).

Make healthy changes. Choose whole grains such as brown rice or whole-grain bread over refined white rice and bread. Avoid French fries and the cheese-stuffed potato and order two vegetables, steamed, or a salad and vegetables. Instead of pasta dishes with cream, opt for those with tomato sauces, which are generally lower in fat and calories.

Be careful with how much wine you drink. If you want a glass, by all means have it. Just do not go overboard. One study found that women who indulged in more than two drinks a day consumed nearly 30 percent more calories. Stick to one glass of wine. A 125g glass of white wine has about 77 calories, red has 85 calories.

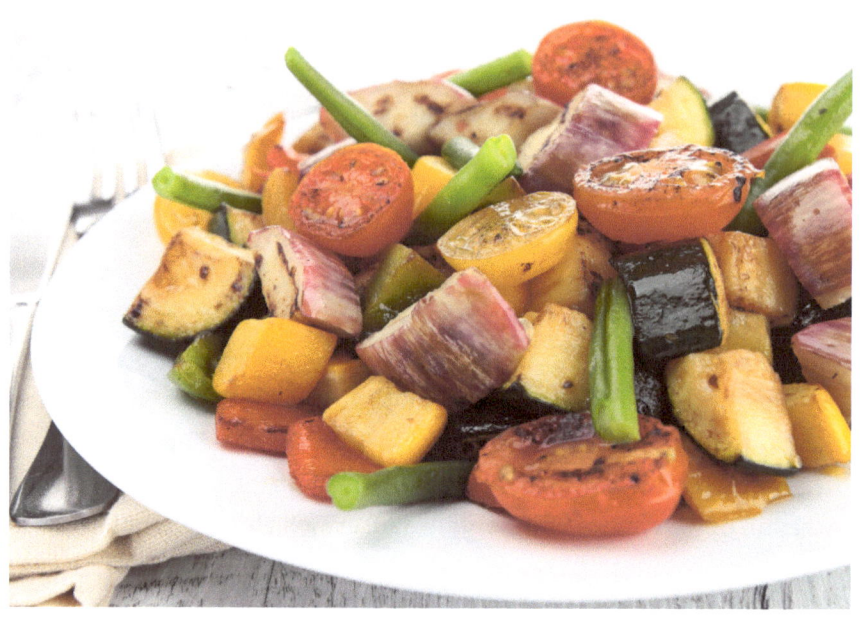

Eat dessert. This is not a joke. Try to deny yourself the chocolate pudding that sounds so delicious and you just might eat something worse (like an entire tub of ice cream) when you get home. The smart strategy is to order one dessert for the table. A few bites should satisfy your sweet tooth. You don't want to share today? Ask for a dish of berries or a small fruit sorbet.

CAN I HAVE PROTEIN SHAKES WHILE ON THE DASH DIET?

The energy used up in making carbohydrate, for example, available to the body as energy compared to the energy used up converting protein to usable energy is substantially different. 100 calories of carbohydrate eaten may make 93 available to the body; 100 calories of protein eaten may make only 70 available. – *See Jequier, "Pathways to Obesity", International Journal of Obesity, (2002).*

Most people gain all of the protein they need from eating a normal diet. Protein shakes provide protein in a particularly easy-to-digest way. Weight trainers need extra protein to build muscle when exercising. The main problem with a lot of these protein shakes is that they also have other ingredients such as carbohydrates and artificial chemicals to enhance colour and taste.

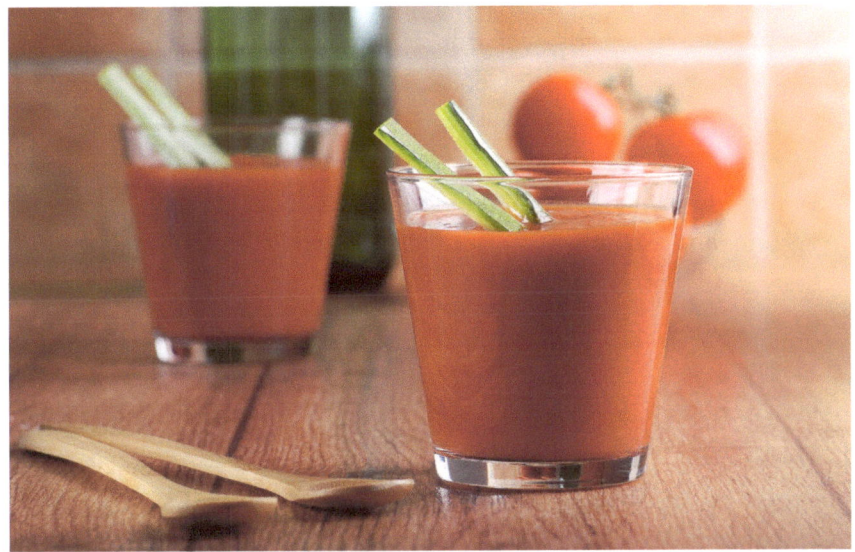

Protein shakes will only bulk your body up when you combine them with exercises that build muscle. That is their purpose.

ONCE I REACH MY IDEAL WEIGHT, CAN I STOP EXERCISING AND DROP THE DASH DIET?

Dieting should be seen in two phases, the first phase is to lose your excess weight, and the second phase is to keep the weight off. When you get to your ideal weight, you need to learn how to eat and exercise without changing your weight. So you can increase what you eat gradually, or decrease the amount you exercise gradually, until you reach a weight plateau that you are happy with. You may find that you still need to exercise, but not as much as you were doing during the first dieting phase.

IF I REDUCE MY EATING STICK TO THE DASH DIET AND STILL DO NOT LOSE WEIGHT, WHAT SHOULD I DO?

Increase the amount of calories that your body burns by increasing the amount of exercise you do. Start going for a jog in the morning, walk or bicycle to work instead of using the car or public transport, use stairs instead of the elevator.

Try a high protein high fat, low carbohydrate diet, by keeping your protein and carbohydrate intake separately and retraining your body to use protein for energy instead of the quick energy you get from carbs.

HOW MANY CHEAT DAYS CAN I HAVE PER WEEK ON THE DASH DIET DIETING?

The short answer is NONE. This might sound hash, but here are some reasons.

If you cheat, your body does not adapt to your new healthy diet. When you drastically change the way you eat, a certain adaptation process takes place. Your body needs to change how it has been metabolising and how you have been burning fat naturally.

If you keep cheating, you will prevent this metabolic adaptation from ever fully completing. Also, when you abandon the standard western diet and start eating more real foods, it can take some time for the sense of taste to adapt.

With time, real foods start to taste much better. If you cheat and eat junk foods frequently, your taste sensations will not adapt completely and you will not be able to experience the same satisfaction from real foods.

You might binge and eat way too much. Some people can binge like there is no tomorrow and ruin a week's worth of dieting in one sitting. It has been known for bingers to eat 5,000 calories in one sitting. That is two days' worth of calories for a grown man and an entire week (or two) of dieting pretty much ruined.

Cheating does not raise metabolism or prevent "starvation mode". The concept of "starvation mode" is largely a myth with no real science behind it and does not really happen until you get to an extremely low body fat percentage. For healthy people trying to stay healthy or lose a bit of weight, cheat meals are unnecessary at best and may be detrimental.

If you are worried about your metabolic rate going down during a weight loss period, lift weights. This is actually proven to maintain both your metabolic rate and your muscle mass.

Those nasty ingredients will never completely leave your body. Trans fats, seed oils and gluten - these nasty ingredients linger in the body for a while and it takes a long time to fully recover from their effects. If you keep eating them, they will never completely leave your body.

HOW MUCH WATER DO I DRINK ON THE DASH DIET?

About 70% of your body is water. You need to take in about 2 litres of water a day to stay hydrated. When you get dehydrated, your body starts to suffer. Your thinking ability deteriorates; you will feel increasingly tired with little stamina. Your mouth and eyes will feel dry. Lack of water can even inhibit a person's workout routine.

Being dehydrated can actually cause you to gain weight. Water helps us to maintain a healthy weight by suppressing our appetite, reducing our body's level of sodium and helping us to maintain muscle tone. Dehydration causes a person to become hungrier, resulting in higher calorie consumption throughout the day.

So ensure you stay hydrated. Drink plenty of fluid every day, water, green tea, coffee. Not soda or beer.

CAN SUGAR MAKE ME TO GAIN WEIGHT WHEN I'M ON THE DASH DIET?

Most western processed food contains sugar to improve the taste. Until recently, nutritionists suggest that people should get only 10% of their calories from sugar, now WHO recommends 5%. Getting 10% equals 13 teaspoons of sugar per day (based on 2,000 calories per day), while 5% equates to 6.5 teaspoons per day! The current average for an American is 42.5 teaspoons of sugar per day!

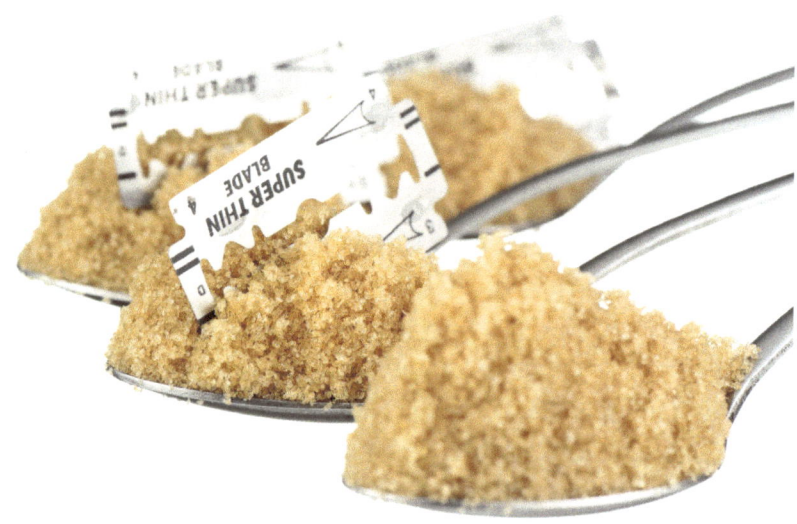

A 12 oz. can of soda, such as Pepsi or Coca Cola, has the equivalent of 10 teaspoons of sugar in it. How many do you drink each day?

See this breakdown of where else we get sugar in our diet:

Percentage Item

10%   Sweetened fruit drinks

5%   Candy

5%   Cake

4%   Ready-to-eat cereal

4%   Table sugar and honey

4%   Cookies (biscuits) and brownies

4%   Syrups and toppings

26%   Prepared foods such as ketchup, canned vegetables and fruits and peanut butter

Another high-sugar category is low-fat products, which may not be as good for your diet as you might believe. Some contain A LOT of sugar to make up for the lack of the fat which often gives food its taste. So the calorie count of the low-fat version of your favourite mayonnaise may not be much different from the full-fat original.

Once you start checking for sugar in the processed foods in the supermarket, you will find it almost everywhere. Sugar is used to add flavour to foods instead of fat. The food industry has done this as a way of getting us to continue to eat what they manufacture.

HOW CAN I GUARANTEE THAT I REDUCE MY FAT BELLY?

Increase the amount of time you exercise. Try doing some squats and dead-lifts to strengthen the muscles in your back and stomach area.

Eat healthy food you cook from scratch. Concentrate on these examples:

**Proteins**: Eat plenty of lean meat, poultry, fish, whey, eggs, cottage cheese.

**Vegetables**: Spinach, broccoli, salad, kale, cabbage.

**Fruits**: Banana, orange, apple, pineapple, pears.

**Fats**: Olive oil, fish oil, real butter, nuts, flax seeds.

**Carbs**: Cut down on your carb intake. Eat brown rice, oats, and whole grain pasta.

**Reduce your alcohol intake**. To lose your belly fat, what you drink is as important as what you eat. A little alcohol from time to time is OK. But forget about losing your belly fat if you drink beer & "alcopops" daily. Beer drinkers always have a pear shape: belly fat and man boobs – especially as they get older. Alcohol also stresses your liver which has to work hard to clear the toxins from your system. This gets in the way of building muscles.

WHAT CAN I DO TO BOOST MY METABOLISM?

As you age you lose about 2-3% of lean muscle tissue per decade. This naturally reduces your metabolism as you get older. To reverse this, you have to work hard to increase your muscle mass by exercising. Take up weight training.

WHICH 5 EXERCISES CAN I DO TO LOSE WEIGHT?

Tai Chi. This is a Chinese martial art that incorporates movement and relaxation, good for both body and mind. It has been called "meditation in motion." Tai chi is made up of a series of movements, one transitioning gracefully into the next. Tai chi is accessible, and valuable, for people of all ages and fitness levels, because classes are offered at various levels.

Swimming. Swimming is almost the perfect workout. The buoyancy of the water supports your body and takes the strain off painful joints so you can move them more fluidly. Swimming is good for individuals with arthritis because it is less weight bearing. Research finds that swimming can improve your mental state and put you in a better mood. Water aerobics is another option. These classes help you burn calories and tone up.

Strength training. If you believe that strength training is a macho, brawny activity, think again. Lifting light weights will not bulk up your muscles, but it will keep them strong.

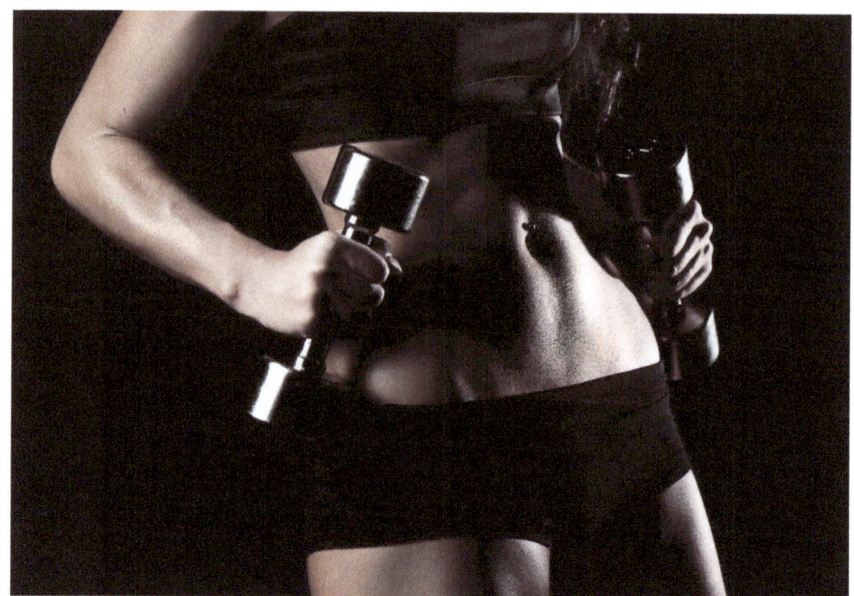

Muscle also helps burn calories. The more muscle you have, the more calories you burn, so it is easier to maintain your weight. Strength training might also help preserve your ability to remember.

Before starting a weight training program, be sure to learn the proper way to do it. Start light with just one or two pounds. You should be able to lift the weights 10 times with ease. After a couple of weeks, increase that by a pound or two. If you can easily lift the weights through the entire range of motion more than 12 times, move up to slightly heavier weight.

Walking. Walking is simple yet powerful. It can help you stay trim, improve cholesterol levels, strengthen bones, keep blood pressure in check, lift your mood and lower your risk for a number of diseases (diabetes and heart disease for example). A number of studies have shown that walking and other physical activities can improve memory and resist age-related memory loss.

All you need is a well-fitting and supportive pair of shoes. Start with walking for about 10-15 minutes at a time. Over time you can start to walk farther and faster until you are walking for 30 to 60 minutes on most days of the week.

Kegel exercises. These exercises will not help you look better, but they do something just as important - strengthen the pelvic floor muscles that support the bladder. Strong pelvic floor muscles can go a long way toward preventing incontinence (involuntary urination) While many women are familiar with Kegels, these exercises can benefit men too.

To do a Kegel exercise correctly, squeeze and release the muscles you would use to stop urination or prevent you from passing gas. Alternate quick squeezes and releases with longer contractions that you hold for 10 seconds, and the release for 10 seconds. Work up to three 3 sets of 10-15 Kegel exercises each day.

WHICH 5 THINGS WILL MAKE THE DASH DIET GUARANTEED TO WORK?

Cut down on the amount of alcohol you drink. Eliminate it totally if possible. Alcoholic drinks contain what are known as "empty calories" and your body has to work hard to get rid of the poison that alcohol is. When it is doing this, it can't digest the food you've eaten to make it work for you.

Exercise more. You don't need to visit the gym. You can cycle or walk briskly around town. Visit the swimming pool regularly.

Eat healthy food. Avoid processed foods with extra sugar in.

Keep hydrated. Drink plenty of water, tea and coffee - at least two litres a day.

Manage your stress. When you are stressed, your body chemistry changes. You may find that you become hungry at strange times and your will power to resist snacks will decline. You may be drawn to unhealthy but easily-available foods, such as confectionary. As much as possible, try not to succumb.

HOW CAN I REDUCE MY FLABBY ARMS?

You need to improve the tone of the muscles in your arms. Take up exercise that will strengthen these muscles, such as swimming or tennis. You could try weight training at the gym as well..

THAT'S A WRAP

If you have read this whole book, you will have read a lot of advice on dieting and exercise. These two things go hand-in-hand when it comes to losing weight. You have to change your whole approach to life to get down to your goal weight, not only change what you eat but be much more active than you might have been before.

It is hoped that at least some of these guidelines will allow you to have success!